SO YOU WANT TO BE A DENTAL HYGIENIST

The Good, The Bad, and The Ugly

The quick guide to helping you

determine if a career in

dental hygiene

will be the career for you.

LISA NITKOWSKI, RDH

CONTENTS

ACKNOWLEDGEMENTS

This book is dedicated to my mom, Irene, and my sister, Jennifer.

Mama, you showed me what the epitome of being a woman means. Your support, strength, and resilience gave me the supreme role model to look up to. Thank you for never giving up on me and knowing that I could make you proud.

JenJen, you are the most amazing and brilliant human I know. You are strong, beautiful, and my sounding board. It is because of your help, guidance, and unconditional love that I was able to continue to fight my battles and survive.

Without you both, I would have never realized my dreams or had the courage to go after them.

Thank you for always believing in me. I feel so very blessed to have such amazing women as you for my family. I love you both, unconditionally and forever.

~ Love, Leelee

INTRODUCTION

Dental hygiene isn't necessarily the first thing you think of when you think of healthcare. At least for me it wasn't, but I honestly never really knew or thought too much about it. I usually thought of healthcare involving people with the titles of "doctor" or "nurse" who worked in places like "hospitals". Of course my parents took my sister and I to the dentist and we got our teeth cleaned by the hygienist, but after the appointment was finished I never gave it a second thought.

Dental hygiene is actually a really special profession. I call this profession a hidden gem, which is exactly what I thought when I was first introduced to it fifteen years ago. In fact, I fell into the dental field completely by accident. It all started when I was flipping through the newspaper want ads and saw a listing for a dental assistant. The ad simply stated, "Dental Assistant Wanted No Experience Necessary". I had always been curious about dentistry in the back of my mind and figured, why not find out what this whole thing is about? So I responded to the ad and set up an interview. I was definitely a bit apprehensive as the only working experience I had up until that point was in retail. The day of my interview came, and dressed in business casual attire with a big nervous smile on my face, I walked in with my resume in hand. The dental office was busy that day, and of course, I was a bit anxious to sit down with the doctor, as I had no idea what to expect. The manager retrieved me from the waiting area and walked me back through the door where I began looking around the octagon-shaped building and peered into the operatories where the other staff members were working. We finally came to the dentist's personal office, where I proceeded to take my seat across from his. He began to describe the job duties to me and told me a little bit about himself, how the office was run, and what would be expected of me. He then proceeded to ask me questions about my life, where I grew up, and what my previous working experience was. Then he finally asked the question, "So why do you think you'd be good for this job?" I responded with complete honesty, "Well, I have no experience in this whatsoever, but I am a hard worker and a fast learner, and I can get the job done," and he hired me.

This doctor took a chance on me. Honestly if he hadn't, I am not sure that I would have pursued this field a second time, I am not sure where my path would have led me to. As young as I can remember, my passion was to be in law enforcement. Only after embarking on my college career did I realize that law enforcement was not going to be a good fit for me. However, because he did take that chance on me, I was determined to stay true to my word.

Within a short time, he complimented me on my ability to catch on quickly and develop rapport with his long-standing patient base. I was flattered and even more motivated to learn, so I continued to develop my newfound skills. Being artistic, I had always been very good with my hands and creating things, so to me dental assisting was almost like an art class. After some time, I began to take more notice of the hygienists within the practice. They were these amazing women who always appeared happy and optimistic. They were able to come into work every day with a great attitude and still go home to their families at the end of the day with energy left over. They maintained a balance in their lives. A lot of professions I had seen up to that point required people to take their work home with them or left them exhausted, and that was something I never wanted for myself. The hygienists were also adored by their patients. People would get seriously pissed if they weren't able to see their particular hygienist. The relationship between the hygienists and their patients was more than a professional relationship; it was more like they were friends. This intrigued me because it wasn't like in a typical medical setting, such as a hospital, where people seemed more scared or unhappy. Granted, it was a dental office and some people still had their phobias of the dentist, but they were mostly very happy to see everyone. It was different.

I started asking the hygienist's about their jobs and the roles they played. I inquired about their schooling and of course about how much they were getting paid. Two out of the three women I worked with only had their associates degree and did quite well with just that. These women were each making an average of $70K a year! Mind. Blown! You mean I could go to school, earn my associates degree, and come out making that much money? Seriously? Sign me up! Even though the financial gain was one of my motivating factors, it wasn't just that. I liked that you could come into a positive atmosphere, work with your hands, and maintain balance in your life without being overly stressed.

I immediately began looking into the dental hygiene programs available in my state, which at the time was New Jersey. Out of the few schools that offered the hygiene program, there were a couple of colleges that were relatively close to my home, but they each only accepted forty applicants per year. I started to panic a bit as school and book smarts had not always come easily to me. I am the type of person that was born with street smarts and common sense, but I knew if I put my mind to it I could get it done. I was twenty-three years old when I moved back home to live with my mom so I could afford to enroll in school and still keep my job. Moving back home was the best decision I ever could have made for myself, but it also meant a longer, more exhausting day.

After enrolling in school part time while maintaining my full time dental assisting job, my days started at 4:00 a.m. I would get my workout in, shower, pack my breakfast and lunch for the day, drive an hour to work, work my eight-hour shift, drive an hour back, go to class, come home and study and get to sleep by 11:00 p.m. The next day, repeat.

I continued that routine for three years until I was able to complete all of my prerequisites for the hygiene program. I often look back at that time in my life and wonder how I ever did it. But honestly, it's true what they say: if you really want something bad enough, you will find a way; if you don't, you will find an excuse. I found my motivation to keep going. Granted, I was still very fortunate in my situation to have the support of my mom through everything and I realize there are many of you reading this right now who may have it a lot harder. It is still doable. All of our situations are different and we all have our own struggles, believe me, I had mine too. There will always be someone out there that has it a lot harder than you. No matter what your goals and aspirations are for yourself, they are attainable.

Finally, the time came for me to apply to one of the two dental hygiene programs closest to me. All that time of going back and forth, the early mornings, the long work shifts, the shitty pay, the late nights, everything, was about to pay off. Feeling confident, I submitted all of my paperwork. I was super nervous and excited. After waiting for a few weeks, I received my letter from the college. My heart was beating so hard from the sheer nerves and excitement that I started to shake. I had the biggest smile on my face and was already so excited to tell my mom the good news. All I remember reading as I opened the letter was, "Dear Lisa, We are sorry, but we regret to inform you that your application has been denied…" My jaw dropped and my heart sank. As you can probably imagine, I fell into complete shock, then sadness, then anger, and then tears were streaming down my face like a river from the blow I just received. It was heartbreak. I was so hurt and devastated that all I could do was scream every profanity I could think of. I locked myself in my room for a while and felt so completely hurt, disappointed and ashamed. Why ashamed? As I said earlier, school or book smarts were never my strong point, and after all the support my mom had given me, I felt like I had let her down. The one thing I so desperately wanted in this world and the thing I had worked so hard for up until that point was taken from me in mere seconds with a few words on a piece of paper. I mean, how could they!?

There are several forms of heartbreak in this world, but when it comes to your dreams literally crumbling in your hands, something you want so badly, it's devastating. I mean, I couldn't even get my foot in the door! On the same note, I'm also the type of person that if you tell me I can't do something, I'll come back at it a hundred times harder. I'm pretty stubborn that way. After the initial hurt faded, I got pissed and then I got focused. The college I had applied to was a community college that in all honesty, I thought would be easier to get into. Smack me now. The other college that was close to me that also offered the hygiene program was actually my first choice: a well-renowned university which would afford me more admiration and recognition. It was also more difficult to get into which is why I didn't even attempt it since I just automatically assumed that they would turn me down. I went back to my college and spoke with a counselor, and they said that I only needed one more course to fulfill the prerequisites required to apply to that school: public speaking. The sheer thought of speaking in front of people made me extremely nervous: I'm talking sweaty armpits and swamp ass with a face that gets as red as cherry during presentations. I tried to avoid it like the plague. But sometimes, you just have to do what you have to do, especially if you want it bad enough, and that means pushing through those fears. Fast-forward a few months, I completed my public speaking class and surprised myself with how well I did due to an incredible and supportive teacher. I was then able to apply to my first-choice university and was accepted. This time I had tears of joy streaming down my face because I not only pushed through some fears, made my mom proud, and made myself proud, but also it was the start of a new life for me. I was going to be enrolled in the dental hygiene program.

Whatever your reason may be for wanting to become a dental hygienist, your search has led you to this book. You picked this book up in the hopes of getting a little more clarity about whether this field is a good fit for you. Just like I probably would do if I were back in your shoes right now, I would try to see if this career is all that I hope it will be. You want to figure out if the schooling, time, effort, money, what happens after you graduate, and what it's really like to work as a registered dental hygienist (RDH) in the real world is something you can actually see yourself doing. Whether you are just starting your college career, or this will be your second or third career change, this book will help give you a look into the good, the bad, and the ugly parts of this profession.

Every career has these three categories and it would definitely be something I would be looking into if I was seriously contemplating this path. I can honestly tell you that dental hygiene is not for everyone, and for others, it may be the perfect fit. Of course, there is no better teacher than experience, so I will do my best to share with you everything I have learned, gone through, and observed in my career and from the many other hygienists I have met over the years. I promise to give it to you with brutal honesty, warts and all. As you make your way through the pages to come, I encourage you to underline, highlight, and take note of key components that are important to you. You may even consider making a chart with the three sections and writing down below each section the points that struck you the most.

This is your life, after all, and you deserve nothing short of absolute happiness. That is what I ultimately want for you. Time is our most precious commodity and it is the one thing that we cannot make more of or get back, so I am not here to waste it. I have attempted to make this book as short, sweet, and to the point as possible. When it comes to deciding on your career and future path and thinking about all of the time, effort, and work you will spend on your schooling, you should feel confident and as well-informed as you can be in your decision. We spend so much of our time working that we should at least give ourselves the very best chance we can to pursue something that will indeed make us happy and fulfilled.

I am one of those people who believe that everything happens for a reason. There's a reason you settled on this career path. It is my hope that I can help you figure out your "why." It is my hope that I can help you make the right choice for you and your life. There may be people who question why you want to pursue dental hygiene. I mean, it's *the dentist*, right? Who likes going to the dentist, let alone working in a dental office? And "Oh my God! Working in people's mouths? Ew!" Actually, I have met more people that love coming in and seeing their dentists and hygienists than don't, let alone the passion that these healthcare providers have for this field. My point is, everyone has an opinion, but the only one that should matter is *yours*. There will be negativity, and you may feel discouragement, but I don't want you to listen to people who have no clue what they're talking about because they actually have no idea what the hell they're talking about! It may seem strange that I am even mentioning something like this but I have seen this firsthand where people who are thinking about dental hygiene begin to second-guess their choices due to the opinions of others who have no relevant experience in dentistry whatsoever. Stop listening to the naysayers and listen to the people - hopefully I'll be one of them - that actually have been in the trenches and have been there.

This book will give you firsthand insight into a profession before you commit to the schoolwork and take thousands of dollars out in student loans. Imagine getting a sneak peak into a possible future you have your goals set on and seeing how things may turn out. It is my belief that most people would take the option to know what might happen and how it would all turn out for them, and if in fact it would be a wise decision.

My purpose in creating this guide is to give anyone interested in this career *their* chance, just as that doctor had done for me when I first walked into his office years ago. As you will come to learn in the following pages, the dental hygiene profession is more than just "cleaning teeth." So if you're ready to learn all about the good, the bad, and the ugly parts of this career to see if this is a right fit for you, let's get started.

PART I

THE GOOD

Let's start with the good stuff. I want to help you realize all the great things about this career - not just what it has to offer you, but also what you can offer it. Your reason for choosing this profession will vary. Dentistry may run in your family or you may have been inspired by a friend or even your own hygienist. Perhaps it was financial motivation or because you want to be involved in one of the fastest-growing healthcare professions out there. Dental hygiene is a rewarding field that allows you to take on the role of a healthcare provider and an educator, all the while helping people become healthier overall. You will also forge friendships and relationships with people that you may never have met otherwise.

Thinking back to the day when I was first welcomed into dentistry, it was then that I started to learn more about the hygienists, what they do, and who they are as healthcare providers. We are indeed *healthcare* providers. Hygienists provide more than clean teeth: we are educators, prevention specialists, professional colleagues, and confidants. We work side by side with our doctors and specialists to custom tailor a treatment plan for each individual patient that will offer the most benefit for their oral health. The patients in the dental practice see the hygienist far more often than they see the dentist, especially when the patient is on a three-, four-, or six-month recall for their appointment. This means we are usually able to develop wonderful, close interpersonal relationships and sometimes even friendships with our patients.

The hygienist is a valued and key player in the dental practice. The doctors and specialists we work with value our opinion when it comes to deciding on how to proceed with a patient's care. We focus on the details they do not. While the doctor comes in and does the exam on the patients, they rely on us to provide feedback on any issues the patient may be having, whether with their oral health status or any changes that are pertinent in their medical history. We examine every millimeter of the mouth, literally. We take measurements of the gums to assess for disease, check for abnormal oral pathology, and recognize teeth that may be in need of repair or any aesthetic concerns the patient may have. We are the first line of defense in battling gum disease. We are the doctor's second set of eyes when it comes to finding something that even they may have overlooked or was not apparent until we got in there and started scaling. The schooling we receive also makes us aware of any systemic health issues that are current or may arise, due to clues found in the mouth that even the patient is unaware of. We are constantly using critical thinking skills and our knowledge base to figure out what may be wrong and how to treat the problem. It's almost like we are detectives: assessing the clues, and finding a solution.

The following sections will discuss in further detail all of the *good* things that you can expect and will come across in this career.

Education

Since you are just at the beginning of this journey to determine if the time, effort, and finances you put into your schooling will be worth it to you, I figured this would be the best place to start. Every school in every state may have different prerequisites for applying to their dental hygiene program. As I mentioned earlier on, for example, one school required me to have public speaking though the other school did not. Some schools will require you to purchase all of your instruments and supplies in addition to your textbooks, and others will include all of your instruments and supplies, aside from the textbooks, in the cost of the tuition. This will vary, as will the general cost of your education.

This section will hopefully give you a little more guidance and insight on the schooling for each level of the dental hygiene degree. The level of schooling you need depends on your personal goals and how far you intend to go in school. Each degree you graduate with will allow for more growth in your career, as in any other profession. How much time you have to dedicate or what your professional aspirations are will dictate what you will be able to do and how you will be able to progress professionally. I'm not going to blather on too much about each degree here, but hopefully you will get a good idea of what might eventually interest you. This may also help you decide if progressing to that next degree will be worth it for you. So here we go!

Associate's. With an associate's degree you will be able to get to work immediately in a clinical setting. This is primarily what I have been talking about as far as connecting with patients and other providers such as dentists, specialists, other hygienists, and assistants. I feel like this is where the real "meat" of the profession is. You will be able to provide a valuable service to your patients and become an invaluable colleague to all those you work with. This is where you will continue to master all of your clinical skills while continuing your education through CEs, continuing education credits, which will be required for you to maintain your license as a RDH. Also, you will be able to gain financially, as the pay rate for hygienists is pretty damn good. The hygiene department of any office is the bread and butter of a practice, and we are compensated quite well for what we do. Of course this varies in the state you work in. But rest assured, you will be able to pay off any student loans in no time.

Bachelor's. Earning a BS or Bachelor of Science degree in dental hygiene will open up a few more doors for you. You will be able to work for companies such as Colgate-Palmolive or Proctor & Gamble doing research for them, just to name a couple. Being able to provide research and feedback in a major company about the products that help millions of people around the world can be incredibly rewarding. Some RDHs also get involved in sales positions with these and other dental supply companies which, along with your background and knowledge in this field, can only boost your credibility. You can also obtain a teaching position with your degree and teach future hygienists and even dental students.

For example, before I even graduated, that was one of the questions a couple of my professors asked me, "Lisa, do you happen to have your bachelor's degree?" I said, "No, why?" They said, "That's too bad! We're asking because we would have loved for you to come back and teach here in the clinic!" Okay, so imagine my surprise when my professors asked me to join them teaching in the clinic! I mean, I hadn't even taken my state board exam yet, so I was honored. Then, honestly, I felt a little disappointed because I didn't have this degree under my belt and I had to turn the opportunity down. So if becoming a teacher is part of your future goals, a bachelor's degree is your next step.

I have known several dental hygienists over the years who have worked in colleges and universities not just teaching other future RDHs, but also supervising dental students in the clinic with all of their dental hygiene procedures. These hygienists are still able to work in private practice when school is out. I truly admire these hygienists, as they share their skills and knowledge to improve those of others, whether they are their patients, future hygienists, or dental students.

Master's. This degree helps you grow not just personally, but also professionally. It allows you to expand all of your accomplishments, your skill, and your knowledge and take it all to a whole new level. Professionally this will boost credibility and give you more business and networking opportunities no matter what direction your career may take you in. You can find more doors opening to you with teaching, research, and public health as well. However, having a master's in dental hygiene will not necessarily improve your pay rate if you work in private practice.

Expanded Functions. In some states dental hygienists are able to provide more than just dental cleanings for their patients. The laws of your state determine how much autonomy you have as a hygienist, including whether you can place a filling for a patient or even have your own practice. You will need to look up the requirements of your particular state and determine your options, as they vary state to state.

As I mentioned earlier, depending on what you plan to achieve with your career and your personal goals, you may have to obtain the next level of education. However, if you feel like obtaining an associate's degree will be just as fulfilling, then go for it. No matter your goals, these degrees, even an associate's degree, are no easy task and will require a lot of study time and hard work. You will be sure to find yourself equally challenged and fulfilled.

Employment Opportunities

Obviously, you would like to know if the degree you are deciding on will get you employed, and quickly. There is nothing more stressful than getting student loans to get a degree only to struggle to find a job so you can pay off those loans. Don't worry! This field has more opportunities than you think!

I'm going to focus more on the clinical setting of work as this is pretty much where most, if not all, of us start our career. To be honest, many positions in either research or education will require you to have some clinical experience when you look to expand your horizons. Besides, you went to school and spent an enormous amount of time working on instrumentation and ergonomics and obtaining knowledge that you're going to want to put to good use. It's important for you to master and expand those skills in a clinical setting because that will only make you more of an asset when you do transition into a research, teaching, or even sales environment.

Temping. Temping is a great way to start out, and I actually encourage you to do so, for a few reasons. You can decide which office you would like to work in, and sometimes you can even set your pay rate for that office. If the office seems like it's too far away from home or you don't like the hours, don't take the gig. You can tell the temp agency which days you are available to work and whether you are seeking a part-time or full-time position. Sometimes the office requesting a temp is actually looking for a potential employee, and if things work well between you, you may be a good fit for permanent employment, and the office can buy you out from the agency. This is actually how I procured my first full-time job in Las Vegas. Three months after I moved to Las Vegas, I didn't have a job yet and was temping and taking whatever I could, until one day I walked into an office and it worked perfectly for both of us.

You will have the opportunity to work in different settings, and sometimes it will be a specialty office that focuses on things like pediatric care or periodontal care. You'll get an idea of different situations without having the worry of being committed to that particular office. Each office, even with a general practice, will offer different experiences. This is your time to pick and choose and figure out exactly what you want, all the while keeping up the clinical skills you learned and worked on while you were in school. It will also help with those first-day jitters of working in a clinical environment for whichever office you do finally settle on. We've all been there, so don't worry!

Private Practice/General Dentist. This is the most common type of practice where the majority of working opportunities are. Most of these will be smaller private practices that will have maybe one or two doctors and a staff ranging anywhere from six to twelve employees. These offices can be nice to work in as they typically have a slower pace and the patients feel as if they are coming in to see old friends. In a smaller setting such as this, you are able to develop a close rapport with your patients. There is also a lower turnover rate with employees, and you have the opportunity to gain new friendships at work. These offices tend to be more close-knit and provide the patients with a more relaxed environment.

Specialty Practice. There are specialty offices such as pediatrics, periodontics, or orthodontics. Within a general practice, you may come across all of those specialties. However, when you work for a specialized practice, you will fine-tune skills and learn a few extra things along the way. For example, I used to work in a pediatric office, and the skills I learned for helping kids in the dental office became extremely important and valuable. One thing you will come to find is that many people, primarily adults, have a phobia of the dentist due to childhood trauma they previously encountered with a dentist or even dental hygienist. Working in pediatrics, I learned just how imperative it was to make that child's first visit fun and memorable. Kids are just little adults; they are just more vocal about their feelings. It wasn't always easy, and I definitely suffered a few bites along the way, but ultimately, it taught me some great techniques to help not just kids, but the adult population as well. You would be surprised how universal those methods can be, especially when treating a phobic adult.

Corporate-Based Dental Offices. These are still, in essence, private practice. The corporations which own these offices assign a doctor to head up the office and instill financial goals within the practice. These corporations have a lot of incentives that a lot of smaller, private practices honestly can't or struggle to afford. They supply their employees with 401K plans, full health insurance benefits, disability insurance, and paid continuing education credits along with paid vacation, holidays, and sick leave. Due to the large amount of capital these companies have access to, they are capable of doing a lot of good in local and international communities, serving those in need.

The one company I worked for would set aside a day where the dental practice would pick a few local charities and causes and provide free dental care for those who couldn't otherwise afford it. Treatment included free prophylaxis (dental cleaning), scaling and root planing (deep cleanings), fillings, crowns, bridges, periodontal treatment, and extractions. The staff members would come in and work pro bono to provide these services. Staff included front desk, managers, assistants, hygienists, dentists, and specialists. The office would also provide free beverages and a hot meal for the patients that day. It truly was a great cause and a wonderful experience. Although it was a lot of hard work, the appreciation we all received from the patients was priceless.

The international service opportunities available to the employees of the company allowed them to volunteer their time and travel abroad with a service organization for a true life-changing experience helping those in impoverished countries. The education and knowledge that was brought was invaluable to those who otherwise do not have access to dental care. Furthermore, the organization partnered with a charity there that was able to bring clean, safe drinking water to the communities.

Moving to Another State? No Problem. The beautiful thing about having a dental hygiene license is that even if you graduate in one state, there's nothing stopping you from applying for another state license elsewhere should you decide to move. We can work anywhere! One thing you need to know is that you ***will*** need to obtain another dental hygiene license for that specific state. Depending on the amount of time that has passed since you initially took your state board exam out of hygiene school, you may need to take another clinical state board exam, pass a background check, take a jurisprudence exam, and so forth. All of this varies from state to state, so be sure to do your research. I attended a dental hygiene program in New Jersey, and after a few years, I decided to move to Las Vegas. I was able to obtain my hygiene license in Nevada after submitting all required paperwork and taking a jurisprudence exam along with a few other items. The process was a bit costly and took approximately two months to complete, but now I hold active RDH licenses in both New Jersey and Nevada.

In this field, as with other healthcare professions, you truly can go anywhere. You just need to obtain the necessary documents and take any additional tests to receive the necessary license. I highly encourage you to do the research and call the state board of dentistry in the state you are moving to for more specific information, so you are as well informed as possible. I made sure to have my RDH license in place prior to moving to Nevada, as I was not sure how long the process would be, and I was glad I did. I had heard about another hygienist who also did a cross-country move, and her application for her dental hygiene license was not approved *after* she had already moved out to Nevada. I do not know the specifics of her particular situation, so I cannot comment on that. However, this is a big reason why I emphasize securing your license prior to moving to another state, if possible. Many states also have something called *reciprocity*, which may make it easier for you to obtain licensure in another state, but again, depending on where you are and where you want to go, this will vary.

Military/Government. A few years ago I was sent an offer to apply for a position to work at the Marine Corps Base Kaneohe Bay Branch Health Clinic in Hawaii. The email was sent out to every hygienist in the United States who met specific requirements: graduated from an accredited institution, active hygiene license, and at least three years of experience. I was so excited I inquired about the position by responding to the message as soon as I could after work that day. However, it was not surprising to me that it had been filled almost instantly. I decided to share this section just to show you that the military is another way you can provide your services to our nation's finest should this avenue be of interest to you.

Your Colleagues

As a collective, the people that work in this profession are incredible people. Every single hygienist I have been fortunate to get to know has been nothing but supportive and encouraging: a shoulder to lean on, a sounding board for advice, and a resource for information. There is something about having others who can relate to what we do. We all have good days and bad days, and when we have questions, we know we are asking the right people.

When you are a hygienist, you are also an important colleague. Without us, a dental practice would fail. We are an asset. We are the true backbone of a dental practice. A dentist can only handle so much with the restorative and aesthetic treatment they need to do, and would not be able to focus on providing the proper preventative care and attention to detail that we give to our patients. That's why our doctors rely on us. As a hygienist, you are indeed indispensable.

Your Patients

The people that become your patients are pretty special. You get to meet people from all walks of life, backgrounds, and cultures. They all come with a story. Something that is equally as important than caring for your patient's oral and overall health, is developing their trust in you. This is critical. People can be really self-conscious about their mouths. It's going to be part of your job, but also your part as a good-hearted human, to reassure them and make them feel safe and secure. I have had several patients over the years whose trust I gained, and they have really opened up to me. I have seen their transformations both in their mouths and their self-confidence. I can honestly say that it touches me deeply when they show me their excitement and gratitude. I've literally been brought to tears before when I've seen a positive change in one of my people, because it does mean something. That is a huge part of what keeps me motivated to continue to do what I do. You see the change. You see *them* change. Then *you* change and continue to get better both personally and professionally.

I've never taken a conventional approach to my patients. I have always been very real and direct with them. Patients don't want to be preached to, and the last thing you want to do is make them feel bad about themselves and even more self-conscious about their mouth. People are actually really sensitive about their mouth. Whether they are noticing an odor or they simply don't like the appearance of their teeth or gums, it can be difficult for them to open up to a complete stranger.

Think about it if it was you. Let's say that you went in for an appointment to a doctor's office and had concerns about a bump you noticed on your face. The last thing you want to hear is, "Holy hell, why haven't you gotten that looked at before? Do you realize how bad this could be? Why didn't you get that looked at sooner? What the hell were you thinking letting this go for so long?" Right. Not only would that make you feel awful, but also now you'd be terrified and it would be highly unlikely you'd go back to that doctor, or any doctor for that matter, at least for a while. The last thing you want to do is traumatize or add trauma to someone who is already fearful, which in turn will prevent them from ever getting the help they need. By developing this trust with people and giving them the sense that they can open up to you, you can learn more about them and what's really going on.

For example, I had a case regarding a nineteen-year-old girl. Her mother had brought her into the office for a cleaning as usual. The rest of the staff were already quite familiar with this family as they had been long-standing patients. However, it was the first time I was seeing her. After getting through the dental-related questions - "Have there been any changes to your medical history?" and "Is anything bothering you?" - I proceeded with a little small talk and tried to get to know her. I asked her if she had any plans for the summer, what she was studying in college, and so forth.

As I was doing her cleaning, I noticed some erosion on the back side of her teeth. Erosion on the backside of someone's teeth is usually the result of acid getting into the mouth from the stomach and eating away at the enamel. Enamel is literally the hardest substance in the human body, and it takes quite a bit of acid to cause this to happen. Looking over her medical history again, I saw nothing mentioned about acid reflux. A lot of people are unaware that they even have acid reflux. This goes back to what I was saying about looking for clues in the mouth for systemic issues with the patient that they may not even be aware of. So about a half hour or so into her appointment and after getting to know her a little bit, I asked her, "Do you have any kind of acid reflux going on?" She responded, "No, why?" and I said, "Because you have some erosion going on on the backside of your teeth." She then asked me what that was, and I explained that it was a result of acids coming up from her stomach and going into her mouth and that it generally happens over a period of time. She became quiet for a moment and looked down. She then turned and looked at me and nervously said, "I'm bulimic." She had been purging any food that she had been eating for years. My heart went out to her, and I proceeded to try and talk to her to reassure her of how incredible she already was. We chatted for a little while, and she gave me a hug thanking me for being there for her, even if just for that moment.

Her mother was aware that her daughter was seeing a new hygienist, me, that day and had informed the whole office not to tell me about her daughter's bulimia. I was livid. The mother wanted to keep all of this a secret for whatever reason. Maybe she thought I wouldn't understand. Maybe she thought I would judge her daughter and that she was protecting her from criticism. Maybe she was ashamed that her daughter was suffering from this disease. I honestly never found out her reasoning, but despite all of that, I still found out about the bulimia. I felt that because she failed to tell me about her daughter's condition, she failed her daughter even more. Concealing the problem only leads to more problems. It was my feeling in that moment that her daughter just needed someone to talk to, and by showing her a little compassion and by giving her the time and an ear to listen, she was grateful. What the mother failed to remember was that dental hygienists are still healthcare providers and we have nothing but the best interest of our patients at heart, whether it has to do with their mouth or otherwise. In this case, it was the girl's emotional well-being that needed far more attention that day.

Like I said, trust can be a hard thing to develop when you are just meeting someone for the first time, whether personally or professionally. But once you get that "in" with your patients, it's priceless. I personally love connecting with people and learning about them and their story, their background, where they came from, and who they are. I feel so blessed to have met so many people from all over the world. We all have a story to tell, and when you start to share in their stories and they begin to share in yours, it's just awesome.

This is something that I feel hygiene as a healthcare profession offers you that many others may not. It's all about the connection. We are afforded the time and opportunity to connect with people, find out what their goals are for their oral health, and learn about who they are as people. We get to see the same people consistently every few months, over time, and our relationship with them deepens.

Don't be surprised if there are days when you are acting more like a therapist than a hygienist, because some people just want to talk about what is bothering them. I have had many patients break down in front of me because of personal things they were going through. This is because they felt safe enough to open up to me and be free with their emotions.

When you create this sort of environment, safe and nurturing, then you will see a whole new side to your people, and maybe even yourself. To me, this is one of the most amazing experiences you can have with another human being.

Work/Life Balance

I can honestly say that this is one of those professions where you can go to work and not bring it home with you. There are no papers to grade and no cases or presentations to get ready for the next day, unless of course you pursue a teaching position. Everything you need is already within you. Everything you need to work with, aside from a pair of loupes - more on these later - is already at the office. In hygiene you can even determine what kind of schedule you want. You can work as much or as little as you like. If you're only looking for part-time hours because you need to be home with your kids certain days, that's available. If you want to work six days a week and stack the cash, you can do that too. Just be careful of burnout! If you don't want to commit to a particular schedule and only want to work Mondays and Thursdays or Tuesdays and Wednesdays, or even just work one day a week, that's an option too! You can always call a temp agency and let them know your availability. You have a lot of control when it comes to deciding your schedule. Obviously, the office hours of the individual dental practices will vary, but I think you understand what I'm saying. The opportunities and the schedule you want are out there, you just have to seek them out.

As you can see, hygiene is a pretty well-rounded field. The opportunities for work are many, and it is super versatile. Even with an associate's degree you can make a very good living and provide for yourself and your family. You will be able to spend the holidays with your loved ones and not worry about preparing any kind of presentation or case for the following week. The other hygienists you meet will be just as excited to meet you as you are to meet them. There are also several dental hygiene forums on Facebook and other social media platforms where you will be able to connect with and ask other hygienists for advice or guidance. I personally love these platforms because you gain feedback from hygienists with different backgrounds and experiences. We all have something to offer one another.

We also have a professional organization called the ADHA, American Dental Hygiene Association, which supports the role of the dental hygienist, promotes and broadens career paths, and even provides continuing education. Membership to the ADHA is something that is offered to you once you are ready to graduate with your first degree in hygiene. Are you ready to start your journey yet?

PART II

THE BAD

As you may already be wondering, this is where I start to talk about the things that may not be all rainbows and butterflies. Every profession has a little bit of a dark side. The side that no one really likes to talk about, especially when you are contemplating moving forward in a profession and are about to put in some serious study time and shell out some serious cash for those loans. This is where I will go over some of those things, not to deter you from this career path, but more or less to inform you of issues that may potentially come up. With this information, you can decide if these are things that you can deal with. I told you at the beginning of this book that I would be brutally honest when it comes to talking about this field in its entirety, and I meant it.

Let me start with this: I feel it is important that you remember who you are and who you want to be in your role as a Registered Dental Hygienist. You have taken on the role of a healthcare provider. It's an important and serious role, and you should think about what you want to achieve in it.

What inspires and motivates you to provide the service you have set out to do in your community? What brought you to this decision? I want you to seriously think on it. I'm asking you to think about these things because there will be days where you will get so frustrated that you want to scream, and days where you will go home and cry about your day. I am not kidding when I say that every hygienist has had those days, this one included. How you respond to certain situations will stem to who you are because it boils down to morals, values, and ethics. Let's dive in.

Working Environment

I have personally worked in every role in the dental office aside from being the dentist. A lot of hard work goes into every part. The front desk is always busy with scheduling patients, billing, verifying insurance, confirming appointments, and making sure things move smoothly throughout the day. The dental assistants are constantly running through the office: setting up for patient procedures, assisting their doctor effectively and efficiently, taking on emergencies, clearly communicating between the doctor, patient, and front desk about the next step in treatment, and helping hygiene if they can. Basically, it's a lot of grunt work. Those of you who have experience in dental assisting know that it can be a very stressful job with a lot of work and not so much pay. Here I will begin to discuss some of the issues you may come across with these potential team members.

Your Boss/Dentist. You will have a boss, and sometimes that boss will ask things of you that you may not be completely comfortable with. I am happy to report, however, that these incidences are few and far between. Most of the time your boss/doctor will be super supportive and understanding and will be open to discussing any concerns you may have.

Hygiene Divas. Oh yeah, they are out there and do not turn into one of them! We may have come from different backgrounds, but when we start off in hygiene, we all start with just learning how to hold a scaler in our hand. Just because you start making more money and start buying yourself the fancy clothes and car and designer bags, it does not make you any better than any other team member. Don't be cocky. It's tacky, and no one will want to work with you or put up with the attitude you bring. I have heard of hygienists throwing things at assistants or bossing them around, refusing to clean their rooms or help in the lab with sterilization or office duties in general. You'll be writing your own ticket and will be fired as fast as you got hired.

Office Managers/Front Desk. Sometimes the front office just doesn't understand how hard our job can be. They don't always know all the terminology or what is required for the treatment we are providing our patients. Honestly, they aren't supposed to know what you know, just like you aren't supposed to know everything about the patient's insurance, the type of coverage they have, or their co-pay. It works both ways. Still, because they don't always know, I feel like many of them diminish the weight of the procedure. If a patient is scheduled for a *prophylaxis* or *periodontal maintenance* or even a *scaling and root planing*, they will simply call it a "cleaning" and diminish the weight of the procedure. That may result in the patient not placing much value in what they are having done. For example, if you go to a hairdresser and tell them you want a "haircut" but don't explain the type of haircut you want, it can be disastrous. A light trim off the ends is a far cry from a buzzcut. See what I'm saying? There are differences in the types of treatment we offer our patients, and those should be explained thoroughly, by you, to them. If need be, explain it to your front desk.

Dental Assistants. Dental assistants have a hard job. If you have worked as a dental assistant prior to beginning your hygiene career, you know what I'm talking about. Assistants already have a lot on their plate. I had six years of dental assisting experience prior to starting my dental hygiene career, and I completely value these team members. However, I have also come across some assistants who are just bitter and for whatever reason, have a problem with the hygienist. Understanding that these team members work hard, I have always tried to do what I could to help them between treating my own patients. However, sometimes no matter what I did, they were still negative and had an attitude toward me and any other hygienist in the office.

You will run into these types as well. I can tell you that if someone has an issue with you right from the beginning, it really has nothing to do with you. They are projecting whatever insecurities and personal issues they have onto you and possibly others, even patients, and are simply not happy with themselves. Perhaps they *really* are just unhappy; you never really know and it would be unfair to assume anything even if they do come off as having a chip on their shoulder. Should you ever come across an assistant like this, try having a professional and private chat with them to gain an understanding of what is really going on. If that doesn't change anything, then approach your dentist directly about the situation. Sometimes it will take a meeting of everyone involved - you as the hygienist, the assistant, and the doctor - and sitting down to discuss the issues to gain a bit more clarity and find a solution to the problem.

If there's one thing to remember whether during the course of your career or in life in general, it is always best to keep the lines of communication open rather than letting things build up until it has gone too far. So speak up!

Your Schedule

School. You are on the clock. Your whole day is set up around your schedule, and it is important that you stay on time and on track. When you first start practicing your clinical skills in the clinic in hygiene school, it is honestly not a true, or realistic representation of real-world experience.

In school, they will allot you approximately two and a half hours to work on the fundamentals in the clinic. This will include all of your data collection: reviewing medical history, describing the patient's gums in regards to their color, appearance and any inflammation observed, and oral pathology. You will note any existing treatment in the mouth as far crowns, fillings and so forth, and proceed to obtain measurements of the patients gums to assess for periodontal disease. At this juncture, you would then have a professor come and check what you have gathered, and if all looks good, then you can move on to the scaling of *one* quadrant of the mouth. Depending on your patient's classification and how much tartar is present in their mouth, this can take you more than just one, two and a half hour session, for that one quadrant. This is not unusual especially when you are just learning and getting the hang of things. Trust me, we've all been there!

Reality. When you are finally out in the real world working in private practice, you will generally be given anywhere from forty-five minutes to an hour to do everything for one patient: update medical history, take the patient's blood pressure, take the radiographs if the patient needs them, collect data, scale, polish, floss, discuss home care instructions, and answer any questions the patient may have. Now you need to wait for an exam by the doctor and you cross your fingers and pray the doctor does not leave you waiting for too long, or worse, forget that you even asked for an exam! It happens. After that, you'll need to clean up and break down the room and set it up for your next patient.

Not all recare appointments are created equal. Some patients' tartar buildup will be heavier than others', and some will be lighter. Some patients will show up on time, and others will mosey on in twenty minutes late. Depending on the office you are working for, they may have a policy in place to reschedule those patients after a certain point to help keep you on track. Or, you may still be required to see that patient and you will end up falling behind for the rest of the day. If the patient ends up running late and you are still required to see them, it obviously isn't a good situation for you because it can put the rest of your schedule behind and leave you in a domino effect of unhappy patients who do arrive on time for their appointments. This leaves you in an unfortunate predicament where you are left apologizing and trying to make it up to the next disgruntled patient.

Accelerated Hygiene. Some offices will do something called *accelerated hygiene*. This is where you are double-booked all day, seeing a patient every half hour while having a dedicated hygiene assistant to help you with seating your patient, taking any needed radiographs, polishing and flossing your patient, and flipping your room. You will have roughly thirty minutes per patient to come in and provide the required services. It is possible to see upward of ten to twelve people per day this way, perhaps more depending on how long your shift is. You are still required to probe and scale the patient and discuss any pending treatment in the patient's chart, discuss and recommend any additional services that may benefit the patient, such as fluoride or laser or any other periodontal medicament, and discuss any questions or concerns the patient may have. You have to accomplish all of this while watching your time. It can get overwhelming at times.

This will all come down to the office you work in and whether or not you feel comfortable working in this way. It's your license, your body, your work ethic and your mind, and you don't want to lose any of those. At the end of the day, you want to work somewhere that you will be happy, valued, and appreciated. You don't want to end up feeling drained at the end of your workday, because this can quickly lead to burnout. Everyone is different and content in different environments. Not every office will be for you, so make sure you have a clear vision of how you want to work and an understanding of what the doctor expects of you and what you will be required to do. Don't just take anything, just to have a job somewhere. There are far too many dental offices out there for you to just settle. Instead, find one that is a good fit. Even after you begin working in a new office, there may be a ninety-day probationary period in which the office watches you and how you interact with their patients and evaluates your work ethic and clinical skills. However, keep in mind this is also the time for you to flip it and evaluate the office to see if it is a place you can see yourself working for the long run.

Your Patients

It's true that you meet some truly amazing people in your career. But I won't even pretend that you won't run into some people that won't want to make you pull your hair out. Regardless, these are your people. You are responsible for helping, treating, educating, and caring for them. I know you may be wondering why, then, this part is in the "bad" section. Well, to be blunt, not all patients are excited to see you. Don't get me wrong, the majority of people you see are great. It's just like life in general: there are people you click with and others you don't. When you add the element of *the dentist* to it, you tend to see a few more people that *aren't* happy to see you, and they'll make sure you know it. This is not a reflection on you as a person, this isn't personal. They are reacting to prior experiences they have had. Dentistry and the care that was given years ago was not as gentle or proactive as things are now. Patients were used to associating pain with the dentist. These days it is more about prevention and education. People fear what they don't know. It's going to be your job to educate them and help them feel comfortable and confident when they are in your chair.

Some people will come into your room and from the first second they'll let you know how much they hate the dentist and aren't happy to be there. This was exactly the case with one man in particular who said those exact words to me. I was reading over his chart and as the assistant brought this gentleman into the room and sat him down, all I heard was, "Just so you know I'm not very happy to be here!" I didn't even get a chance to say *hello* to this guy! My first thought was *Okay…. What the hell?* So as I turned my attention away from the computer monitor and looked at him, I took a chance and pulled out my best British accent and said, "Would you feel better if I talked to you like this?" The man smiled and responded, "Yeah! It would!" And I proceeded to speak to him in that fumbled British accent for at least half the appointment. We got a good laugh, and granted, I don't recommend trying this approach with everyone, but I took a chance and it worked for that guy.

Another issue you may come across is people questioning why you need to know about their medical history. *You're not a doctor! Why do you need to know that? Why are you taking my blood pressure? What do you mean I need to premedicate before my appointment; it's just a cleaning!* This is another area where you will have to educate your patients. A lot of information has come out over the years about the mouth-body connection. Your mouth is the closest thing to your head and your heart. There have been several cases where people have died due to an infection that occured in the mouth and had spread to another part of their body. There was an article in the newspaper a few years ago about a twelve-year-old boy who passed away from a tooth infection that had spread to his brain. The boy's family did not have the means to pay for the simple tooth extraction and antibiotics needed to treat the issue. This is an extremely sad and unfortunate situation that may have been prevented only if there were a few factors that could have been helped: the boy's family having access to affordable care, and knowledge for the parents so that they may have been given the information and resources in treating this problem as quickly as possible.

During your time in the dental hygiene program, you will learn the importance of the patient's overall health and the many things you can do to help keep them safe, whether they are happy with you at the time of the appointment or not. The patient's overall health is far more important. Keeping them safe, even if they don't want to hear it - and some will yell and battle with you about it - is the priority. I have literally told patients, " I can tell you what you want to hear or what you *need* to hear." I cannot stress patient education enough to you. It is what I base this entire career on. If your patient doesn't know what something is and/or why something needs to be done, it's your job to explain it to them thoroughly and without a lot of jargon. They don't want to hear a whole bunch of fancy terminology. Explain things as if you are talking to a child. If you understand your subject well, you will be able to explain it to them successfully and thoroughly, and won't leave them scratching their head and turning to the internet for more information. You just never know what they might find. In fact, it may cause an already anxious patient additional anxiety if they are already fearful. Educate! Educate! Educate!

You will occasionally have difficult patients who are challenging to work on, and I am not referring to how heavy their tartar buildup is. Some patients will state that they cannot lie back all the way in the recommended supine or semi-supine position, which means you will have to adjust and adapt to that patient. To spare your neck, back, and the rest of your body, you'll most likely have to stand up for their appointment and practice some old-school dentistry. Other patients won't cooperate no matter how much you try to get them to turn to you or open their mouth a little wider because you're already having a hard time seeing inside that little dark hole that is their mouth. Some patients will gag if you come anywhere near their mouth, leaving you scratching your head as to how they are able to put food in there?

Some patients will be pretty high maintenance when it comes to how *they* want their appointment to go. They can't be leaned back all the way. They need a pillow for either neck support or back support, or both. They need to hold the suction. They want to hold a mirror to see what you are doing. They start texting on their phones over your light space, or worse, take a phone call. You've barely put the mirror in their mouth and they say you stabbed them. They are more interested in having a conversation with you due to all the talking they seem to be doing rather than moving forward with their treatment. They talk to you while you still have instruments in their mouth, or worse, when your fingers are in there and they end up biting you. They *don't* want you to use the ultrasonic scaler on them. They *do* want you to use *only* the ultrasonic scaler on them. They need to use the restroom prior to their appointment and decide the perfect time to go is when you call them back even though they came to their appointment early and had plenty of time to do their business beforehand. They decided to eat a five-course meal prior to their appointment and, of course, didn't have time to brush.

These are just some of the issues that have come up over the years, and not just from my own experiences, but for hygienists from all over. It might be somewhat comical to read about it, but when you start to experience these things for yourself, you'll most likely feel pretty annoyed. You've been warned! It doesn't happen often, but it will happen. Warts and all, remember?

Documentation

Document. Document. Document. This is another critical topic that you will learn about in hygiene school. The patient's chart is a legal document. This isn't necessarily a "bad" thing, but the only reason I put it under this section is that the patient charts are now being done on a computer, whereas just a few years ago they were physical charts and you had to write all of your notes and findings by hand. Although the advancements in technology are wonderful, my concern is that providers are getting lazy with their note-taking. I have seen far too many patient charts where the previous provider had just copied-and-pasted their previous notes with no clear description of their findings or any verbal medical history updates that were made. This is my biggest pet peeve. There was an incident where I had to approach a hygienist about a patient that she had previously seen and they were scheduled with me for a scaling and root planing. There was no documentation noted at the time of her appointment with this patient, nor was there any perio charting completed that would support the diagnosis and need of this patient requiring the scaling and root planing. This was very frustrating to come across as I had to start from scratch and treat the patient as if they were brand new to the office and determine if this would be the proper treatment for that patient after reviewing my findings with the dentist.

You literally cover every millimeter of a patient's mouth. You are required, by law, to document everything you see and take measurements, note any unusual oral pathology, update the patient's medical history as we have already covered in the previous section, note the patient's chief complaint, and especially the state of their oral health and the status of their periodontal disease. Periodontal disease is the number one thing patients file lawsuits for against their dentist and/or dental hygienist if not properly diagnosed and documented. This is why I cannot stress enough that the notes you take and document are of extreme importance. It may end up protecting you and the doctor you work for. As for further protection, I would suggest you obtain malpractice insurance just in case you do get a sue-happy patient. You worked hard for your license, you need to protect it.

Exposure

If you haven't guessed already, you will be exposed to blood and saliva and whatever else is in the patient's body. The work we do can get pretty messy, and things spray and splatter all over the place. There have been days where I have gotten hit in the head with a flying piece of tartar buildup. I have had blood on my ear. I often wonder what I would look like under a forensic light source at the end of my day. Even though you will be taking and reviewing the patient's history in the beginning of their appointment, you can still come across a few issues.

First, the patient may not be entirely honest with you regarding their history or simply doesn't have much of one because they do not go for regular checkups with their medical providers. Many of them, and I have seen this primarily in the older population, do not remember all of the medications they are taking. Pharmacology is among one of the many subjects you will study within the hygiene program, and you will learn that many of them can have oral side effects. It is important for you to know which medications have these side effects. For example, patients who take a baby aspirin daily may have more bleeding. Obviously, there are far too many medications on the market for you to remember all of them in their entirety, so I would advise that you keep a drug reference book in your operatory or simply look it up and notate it in the patient's chart with your chart note as well as in their medical history.

Second, many patients will question you as to why you are taking their blood pressure. You will hear them ask, "I'm just getting a cleaning, why do you need to take my blood pressure?" You would then explain to them that having elevated blood pressure is not healthy for a patient and may actually prevent you from being able to perform certain services, especially if you will be injecting them with local anesthetic, as this may potentially lead to a medical emergency. You will need to educate and explain all of these concerns and potential issues to them. Some of them will understand and appreciate the caution you are taking, and others will become frustrated and angry. Remember, a "cleaning" is never just a cleaning. Some patients will state that they have a condition called *white coat syndrome* and they only have high blood pressure in the dental office. When you are working in someone's mouth, you are stirring up a lot of bacteria which then could travel to the rest of their body and cause a complication, as we have previously covered. It is important to realize that there is an important link between the mouth and the rest of the body and to inform your patients as well. It is always best to err on the side of caution.

Third, some people will not be honest about their medical history. No matter what a patient writes down on their medical history, you are to treat everyone as if they have something. This all goes back to documentation in the patient's chart and you taking the proper precautions using personal protective equipment, which is regulated by OSHA, the Occupational Safety and Health Administration. This not only protects you but your patient as well. Infection Control will be a continuing education course that you will need to take regularly so that you can stay apprised of any new information.

You will be handling sharp instruments in a slippery environment, and depending on the state you are practicing in you may be allowed to give local anesthetic, which means you will also be handling a needle. Don't worry, you will get all of the training you need to feel confident in handling these instruments! The more you do it, the more confident you will be. Just remember, no matter how many years you are in practice, it is important to always exercise caution when you are handling these tools.

Whether we are discussing your schedule and time management, your team members, patients, or taking precautions with bodily fluids and sharp instruments, please trust that you will obtain the necessary knowledge and training to feel confident to manage all of it. You got this!

PART III

THE UGLY

Dentistry Is Changing

The concepts and methods and the way you treat and care for your patients are still the same. However, when it comes to how this business is being handled, it is changing. I only realized this after I moved out to the West Coast to Las Vegas, Nevada. After I moved out West, I quickly saw that things out here operated much differently than what I had experienced back on the East Coast in New Jersey. I attended one of the best programs for dental hygiene at the time in the state of New Jersey. The teachers were ethical, intelligent, kind, and always a source of support. I still speak to them to this day and know that if I ever need advice on something, they are there for me. After a few years, I decided to move out to Las Vegas for a change of pace, both personally and professionally. I knew I would be able to obtain my hygiene license out there and find work without difficulty, and I did.

Now, before everyone on the West Coast goes into an uproar, I'm not knocking the dentistry out here, as I have seen and worked with some really amazing and incredibly ethical and talented providers. However, the general consensus is that it is more focused on the bottom line. I have never in all my time in the dental field heard so much about the money that was needed to be produced each day as I did after I moved out here. Although I have had some experience in this in a private practice setting as well, such as hearing how much money it takes to flip a room or how much a certain brand of masks or gloves cost, I am more specifically referring to corporate dentistry.

There are corporations popping up all over the place taking over dental care. As a new graduate, they make it sound great. As I mentioned earlier, these corporate-based dental offices are able to provide their employees with a full benefits package, 401K, paid CPR and continuing education credits, holiday and vacation time, and the ability to work alongside specialists such as periodontists, endodontists, oral surgeons, and orthodontists. You are given a contract to sign, and you are told that if you hit certain production goals consistently for the month, you get an additional bonus on top of what you're making. It's a pretty good pitch. That's honestly what got my attention, and being a single female, I had to make sure that I had those benefits in place - God forbid something were to happen to me.

I understand that everyone has a different experience. However, my experience in corporate dentistry is not an isolated one, and there have been several other hygienists that have had a similar experience. Each corporate dental office has a doctor-owner, and they all operate under the same umbrella of the corporation. They all have the same business model to follow and have millions of dollars at their disposal. Honestly, it is quite a brilliant business plan, and I completely respect it, from a business standpoint. However, as a provider, I was less than thrilled with it after I had been working in that environment for some time. I felt that everything was a competition: a competition to do better and try to jam more into my schedule, meaning patients and treatments, and a competition against the other providers in the office. Every day I would go look at the "scoreboard" to see who was hitting their goals. If you hit the goal, you were in the green, if you were almost there, you were in the yellow, and if you were below goal, you were in the red. Nobody liked being in the red. Honestly, it stressed me out. It stressed everyone out. Being a provider in dentistry can be stressful enough without you freaking out about some goal number that some non-clinical staff member set for you!

When I was in hygiene school I was taught to provide good, quality patient care and flawless clinical work. I pride myself in my work and the relationships I forge with my patients. However, in this environment, it was mostly about bringing home the numbers. Everything was rushed, such as doing treatments like four quads of scaling and root planing plus a laser treatment or other localized periodontal medicament in an hour. That is completely abhorrent! One of the several doctors in the practice could come up to you at any time and ask you, "Hey, do you have time for a prophy?", and you would have maybe ten to fifteen minutes before your next patient was set to arrive. You could either say yes and look like a hero and a go-getter and be the best hygienist ever, or you could say no and you could risk looking like a terrible, unhelpful employee to your doctors and management because you know you couldn't possibly provide a proper standard of care to that patient in that short amount of time. It's a vicious game.

In the beginning I was so excited to work in this environment for all the reasons mentioned, but as time went on, management continued to change as did the dynamics of the office. It all became very cutthroat. With each new manager brought a new set of goals to strive for. Doctors, hygienists, and assistants were constantly changing, as the turnover rate was enormous. If a patient came in to see one doctor, there was no guarantee they would see the same doctor at their next appointment, or hygienist, for that matter.

Now, I'm not saying that all corporate offices are like this, but the business model holds firm. Your prime objective is to hit the goal every day. I have known several hygienists who have worked in other corporate offices and absolutely loved their office and their owner-doctor. My office was quite large, and I believe the pressure for that office to outperform was definitely put on the providers, hygienist and doctor alike. It wasn't just me feeling this way. There were several other providers, hygienists, and doctors that would come in, look at their schedule, and either see it packed or not. The providers would all go through their schedules and look for an opportunity to add a service or provide a treatment for their patients that day. It wasn't unusual to see over-packed schedules and the providers still stressing out about not hitting their goal for the day. The stress of hitting your numbers on top of treating your patients effectively was immense. There were many days where I felt less than - not just as a hygienist for not being able to hit my numbers, but also because the office environment made me feel so bad about myself that there were many days I would go home and cry from the sheer stress and anxiety of it all.

Eventually, things got so bad in that office for me that even though they were unable to fault me in my work as a clinician, they attacked my character. The very next day I handed them my resignation. I was always taught to be an ethical provider. In life, I was always taught to do the right thing. So if that meant standing up for what was right and speaking out against unethical expectations, I did. I always promised my patients that I would take care of them and be completely honest with them. I would be their voice. I would be the one they put their trust in because they knew I would hold true to my word and them. I would always have their best interest at heart.

When you work with the public, you have a duty to uphold the very core of what this profession is about, and it's to provide healthcare to your patients. Your primary focus should not be to provide a bottom line for the business. Don't get me wrong, I understand that dentistry is a business just like any other, I *really* do, as I have said this many times before. However, if you do good by your patients, the money will come. I once had a manager approach me complaining to me about not producing enough and not hitting my goals. I told her, "I didn't get into this for the business, I got into this for the patient care." and there was nothing else to be said.

When you embark on this career you are taking on all of the responsibilities of being a healthcare provider. You need to know who you are and what you will and will not put up with. There will be days that test you more than others. The schooling is behind you. It's no longer about learning the skills of proper data collection, ergonomics and instrumentation, you already have them. It will come down to you being able to use your voice, just as I have had to do several times, when you feel things are not right or ethical or when you feel uncomfortable with something. Believe me, the emotional toll and stress you will take on because some non-clinical staff, or even sometimes clinical staff members, are pressuring you about financial goals and gains for their business will be harder on you than your hardest patient. This is your license, but more importantly, this is *your* life. Like I told you in the very beginning, you deserve nothing short of absolute happiness and that is what I ultimately want for you. At the end of the day, you need to do everything you can to protect that.

Body and Health Hazards

This profession has its fair share of risks, and it's more than just getting you fingers bitten by patients. Our hands are our livelihood. Those hands are connected to wrists, arms, elbows, shoulders, necks, your head and your back; I mean, you see where I'm going with this. Every part of your body will be affected at one point or another if you do not practice proper ergonomics within this profession. You would think that sitting all day working on people couldn't possibly be a bad situation. But really, it can get very bad. If you do not do what you can to prevent your body from undergoing multiple traumas, then you will, in fact, endure them over the course of your career, which can lead to more severe trauma, including musculoskeletal disorders and pain throughout your body.

Carpal tunnel is among the most common problems a hygienist will experience, and can force one into early retirement. The constant repetitive motions of our hands and wrists and how we sit over the patient and bend our necks, back, and shoulders affects everything. Maybe it starts out with a little tingling, but if something does not get adjusted, it can lead to numbness in your hands and fingers and lead you to surgery, which also isn't a guaranteed fix. I have known a few hygienists that had undergone surgery to fix their carpal tunnel and instead, it ended their career. I am not telling you all of this to scare you, it is more to inform you and hopefully help prevent you from ever getting to that point. Our career is based on prevention and education. This is my way of informing and educating you so that you can take the proper steps to prolong the life of your career.

There are several things you can do to help prolong the life of your dental hygiene career. You can purchase proper fitting loupes, which are special glasses that are armed with magnification lenses to help reduce the strain on your neck. There are instruments you can purchase for yourself such as ultrasonic scalers and instruments that have sharpen-free technology to alleviate the pressure you need to put on your hands while working on your patients. Special saddle-style chairs that can be adjusted to your body to help alleviate the excess stress placed on you while you are working over your patients. Proper fitting gloves will help avoid constriction of the nerves and blood vessels in your hands. Further, keeping up with a healthy lifestyle will help promote your hygiene career as well as your overall health.

Perhaps you might be thinking, "Well, sure, Lisa, but doesn't the dentist supply all of that stuff for you?" The answer is yes. However, just because they have the equipment in the office, it doesn't mean it will fit **your** body or that the instruments will be adequate. This is not a one-size-fits-all kind of thing. You won't know the types of instruments the office may have or even if they are in good condition. I have come across broken scalers and scalers that have been overly sharpened and are unusable. The other question is if the doctor will be willing to purchase more instruments for you if you need them. Usually the answer is also yes, but depending on how many scalers you're requesting, it may not be feasible. I would suggest that you be reasonable in your requests as these instruments are not inexpensive and order only what you need. You may have to go out and purchase some of these items for yourself if you want to help ensure you are doing everything you can to protect yourself and the longevity of your career and your body. Worst-case scenario, you will end up purchasing these items yourself, and you can write it off as a tax expense.

CONCLUSION

After reading through this book you might be wondering if this career is for you. This is why I strongly felt the urge to attempt to give you the best possible idea of what this profession is all about and how things are beginning to change. You know by now that there is no better teacher than experience. Your experience will vary from every hygienist before you, and every hygienist that comes after you. I promise that I have done my best to give you the brutal truth of the good, the bad, and the ugly parts of this profession in the hope that you will make the best decision for yourself. It is everyone's wish that they could just look into a crystal ball to see if the career they decide on will indeed make them happy. The most honest answer I can give you is this: you won't know until you're there.

It is my belief that healthcare is changing. As you have read in the aforementioned pages, there are quite a few amazing things that you will be capable of accomplishing in your role as a dental hygienist. As you have also read, there are some things that are not ideal about it. Like I said in the very beginning, every career has these three parts to it: the good, the bad, and the ugly. No one profession will be absolutely perfect.

Overall, healthcare is a career path that will bring you a certain level of self-fulfillment and an appreciation for your community. If you want to be able to give back to your community, you will have several opportunities to do so, and this is an exceptional way to do it! This is a very versatile career that you can take anywhere with you. Our roles as hygienists are continually advancing. Technology is advancing, and we will continue to do so as well in our provider role. The compassion you are capable of bringing to others will bring you immense joy and gratitude. Helping others and giving back bring about the most astonishing feeling. In my career in dentistry, my patients have brought me to tears because of the level of gratitude they have shown me for helping them better their oral health and themselves. You *will* make a difference!

There will be days when you are stressed, angry, and so upset that you go home crying, and it will make you question the decision you made in entering this profession. There will be other days where your patient, the one that you've helped, comes back to you and looks you right in the eye and from the bottom of their heart says, "Thank you." When you see that, when you hear that, when they hug you because you haven't just helped them with their oral hygiene, it's because you've helped them on a much deeper level. All of that other shit, even on your darkest day, will make it all fade away. It's because you have formed a real human connection. You could have been an ear for them or a shoulder to cry on. What I have learned is that what people want most in this world is to know that they are being listened to and heard, that you care. You can have the most difficult or phobic patient in your chair, and you have the ability to turn it all around for them. The schooling just teaches you the fundamentals. Everything else is all *you*.

I have made connections with individuals both personally and professionally. I have met people from all over the world who came from different cultures and backgrounds, and each one of them came with a story. It was like a very personal one-on-one interview, and I loved learning about each one of them. I have helped countless people in my career and got to see their transformations firsthand. It truly is remarkable. So, if you asked me whether or not I would go into this profession knowing what I know now, would I do it all over again? Yeah, I definitely would.

ABOUT THE AUTHOR

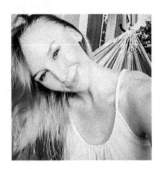

LISA NITKOWSKI has been working as a registered dental hygienist since 2011. She graduated from the University of Medicine and Dentistry of New Jersey - School of Health Related Professions where she learned the importance of patient care and ethical practices. She comes in with a direct, unfiltered and honest approach and now brings her experience and knowledge to others. She has worked from coast to coast and has become passionate to help others find their way.